# The Efficient Nurse

## Master Time Management for Improved Patient Care

# Table of Contents

# Chapter 1. Introduction

Embarking on a mission to help you become the most proficient healthcare professional in your field, our Special Report delves into the crux of "The Efficient Nurse: Master Time Management for Improved Patient Care". This report isn't filled with jargon or confusing technicalities; rather, it distills the essence of time management into bite-sized, digestible knowledge that any dedicated nurse can benefit from. This report showcases inspiring stories, practical tips, and proven strategies of the most effective nurses in the industry, ultimately boosting patient care quality. Become part of the select group of stellar nurses leading the way in efficiency and patient satisfaction. Nurture your passion for nursing, spice up your everyday work life, and let this Special Report guide your transformation into the efficient nurse that every healthcare facility covets and every patient appreciates.

# Chapter 2. The Anatomy of Effective Time Management

The nursing profession is an intricate melding of multiple science and humanities disciplines, steeped in the art of human interaction and driven by the noblest of intentions—care for the sick and ailing. At its heart, however, it is a pragmatic field. A profession unveiled under harsh lights and demanding rhythms; a universe where the clock doesn't stop, deadlines loom, and the roll of challenges is unending.

## 2.1. The Importance of Time Management in Nursing

Time management, in the realm of nursing, translates into essential care practices that can mean the difference between life and death for a patient. Efficient time management can contribute to decreased stress and burnout for the nurse, leading to increased job satisfaction, better patient outcomes, and improved patient satisfaction. If a nurse can administer medications on time, adequately monitor critical condition changes, and facilitate timely discharge dynamics, they potentially save lives, reduce hospital expenses, and enhance the overall patient experience.

In light of these factors, the subject of effective time management in nursing appears to be of grave importance and warrants a thorough exploration.

## 2.2. Understanding Time: Fixed Yet Fluid

On the surface, time is a fixed entity – 60 seconds in a minute, 60 minutes in an hour. However, in the world of nursing, time is fluid. Each patient brings a unique set of needs, conditions, and care requirements, meaning that the same care strategies might not apply to every patient. A nurse must, therefore, adapt their time management to this fluidity, mastering how to prioritize tasks and adapt to unexpected changes.

## 2.3. Prioritization: Sifting through the Sand

Prioritization is the cornerstone of time management. One can imagine nursing tasks as grains of sand, each different in size and weight, yet none visibly more critical than the others at first glance. The nurse's duty is to sift through this sand, selecting the needs that must be attended to immediately. Applying strategies like the ABC (Airway, Breathing, and Circulation) rule from emergency care can help nurses prioritize tasks.

## 2.4. Streamlining Task Management

Once priorities are determined, the next step involves identifying how to perform those tasks efficiently. Streamlining task management often requires eliminating unnecessary procedures, combining tasks where possible, and using technology to aid in routine tasks. Delegate tasks where appropriate. Remember, nursing is a teamwork-based profession, and utilization of all resources, including human resources, is crucial in managing tasks effectively.

## 2.5. Balance and Flexibility

Another vital characteristic of effective time management is balancing planned tasks with flexibility to accommodate unforeseen events. No two days in nursing look exactly the same, necessitating the need for a balance between a structured plan and spontaneity. A well-organized nurse knows the significance of building "buffer time" into their schedule, ensuring they're equipped to handle unexpected challenges without letting their routine tasks suffer.

## 2.6. The Power of Communication

While it's less tangible than the prior points, communication is an integral part of efficient time management. From interacting with patients to liaising with medical professionals and auxiliary staff, nurses need to express their needs clearly, collaborate to solve problems, and maintain a high degree of situational awareness.

## 2.7. Reflect and Adapt

Lastly, effective time management isn't about finding a one-size-fits-all solution. It's about constant reflection, learning from past experiences, and adapting strategies to make improvements. A nurse should regularly reassess their time management strategies, identify areas of improvement, and implement changes as necessary.

Time management is an invaluable skill for a nurse, and mastering it can ensure better patient outcomes, decrease personal stress, and increase overall efficiency. As one journeys down this path, remember that these skills are not innate but learned. It involves continuous growth and adaptation. Superior time management skills in nursing are refined over time, honed through experience, and shaped with an undeniable persistence. Soon enough, you'll find—a well-timed step, a correctly prioritized task—has the potency to revolutionize your nursing practice and elevate patient care to loftier heights.

# Chapter 3. Breaking Down the Efficiency Barriers in a Nurse's Workflow

The art of nursing requires a delicate balancing act between providing quality care to patients and managing a wide range of administrative tasks. Efficiency plays a critical role in this landscape, directly affecting the quality of patient care and the overall patient experience. We'll take a solid look at key barriers disrupting efficient nursing workflow and strategies to break them down.

## 3.1. Understanding Nursing Workflow Barriers

At the heart of each nursing task is a complex nexus of activities we term 'nursing workflow.' Nurses routinely coordinate the confluence of critical-care decisions, patient interactions, coordinating with healthcare teams, documentation, and more. However, obstacles often disrupt this flow, leading to inefficiencies that impact patient care and staff stress levels.

High patient-to-nurse ratios, inadequate staff training or skills, overwhelming documentation tasks, poor technology integration, and inefficient delegation are among primary barriers impacting nursing workflow efficiency. Often these factors lead to time mismanagement, causing delays in care delivery, extending working hours, and heightening job-related stress.

The first step towards dismantling these barriers is acknowledging them and understanding their impact on your workflow and patient care. Realizing you're consistently burdened by extraneous documentation tasks, for instance, allows you to find appropriate solutions such as investing in medical transcription services or seeking more efficient EHR processes.

# 3.2. Prioritizing Tasks

One of the most effective methods for improving nursing workflow is proper task prioritization. Categorizing tasks according to their urgency and importance is crucial. Use the Eisenhower Box, a simple yet effective tool for organizing your tasks into four categories:

1. Urgent and important

2. Important but not urgent

3. Urgent but not important

4. Neither urgent nor important

Spending too much time on urgent but not important tasks can lead to burnout without significant accomplishments. Focus on tasks that align with your role's primary function-caring for your patients.

# 3.3. Streamlining Documentation

Overwhelming paperwork is a significant hurdle. However, today's technology can simplify this. Effective use of EHR systems can not only reduce the paperwork but also make medical records accessible across different departments.

Training is critical here. If nurses aren't familiar with the EHR software, the system that's meant to speed up the process can become another hindrance. So, adequate training on EHR usage to augment your skillset is vital.

# 3.4. Optimizing Team Communication

Communication snags within the healthcare team can cause a ripple effect, hampering productivity and patient care. Implement using effective means of communication like SBAR (Situation, Background, Assessment, Recommendation) to ensure critical information is consistently and accurately relayed.

# 3.5. Delegation and Teamwork

Efficient delegation decreases work pressure and promotes a healthy work environment. A common mistake is to delegate tasks based on job roles instead of capability and capacity. For instance, a nurse mentor could harness the potential of a high-performing team member to help train new staff, freeing up some of their time and nurturing leadership abilities in the team.

Similarly, fostering a teamwork atmosphere where each member recognizes, respects, and plays their part well is vital. Establishing clear roles, collaborating to achieve common objectives, emphasizing open communication, and maintaining mutual respect are key to cultivating a strong nursing team.

# 3.6. Automating and Standardizing Processes

Process standardization and automation is another significant tactic. For instance, define standard processes for routine tasks like changing dressings or administering medication. Minimizing variation reduces time spent on decision making and cuts out mistakes.

By automating repetitive tasks, nurses can focus more on patient care. The implementation of automated medication dispensing systems or patient monitoring devices is an example of technology harnessing to improve efficiency.

# 3.7. Continuous Improvement

Nursing isn't static; it's a dynamic field brimming with constant challenges and enhancements. Staying current is crucial. Participate in regular professional development to sharpen your skills, learn new strategies, and stay updated with technology and best practices.

Each day presents opportunities for improvement; taking stock of what's working well and what isn't will help you adapt your processes to demanding situations continually.

Understanding and breaking down the barriers in nursing workflow are crucial for delivering excellent patient care and reducing stress levels for staff. Through prioritization, effective communication, apt delegation and teamwork, efficient documentation, technology advancements, and continuous learning, you can exploit more opportunities to cultivate efficiency in your workday. Remember, as a nurse, your work plays a critical role in patients' lives, so every step you take towards becoming more efficient has the potential to positively impact a patient's health journey.

# Chapter 4. The Role of Prioritization in Patient Care

As healthcare professionals and especially, as nurses, we deal with high-stake environments where effective time management and savvy prioritization skills are not just advantageous, but necessary for efficient patient care. Prioritization is the heart of being an effective nurse, and mastering this skill can significantly impact patient outcomes, nurse job satisfaction, and healthcare system efficiency.

## 4.1. The Impact of Prioritization on Patient Outcomes

Research indicates that nurse prioritization directly affects patient outcomes, including their overall well-being, recovery times, and satisfaction levels.

When a nurse is able to effectively prioritize tasks, they can ensure that the most critical needs of a patient are met first. This could be administering medication, attending to a rapidly worsening health condition, managing pain, or facilitating fast, effective responses in emergencies.

An expert at prioritization, a nurse can ensure that patient care is directed where it is needed most, not just managing, but actively improving patient outcomes. The concept of "right care at the right time" becomes vividly real, saving time, resources, and, most importantly, lives.

## 4.2. Prioritization and Nurse Job Satisfaction

Prioritization is not just about patients; it affects the nurses themselves, their professional satisfaction, and ultimately, retention in the profession.

In a patient-care setting, the demands on a nurse's time are nearly infinite. Nurses are often juggling a multitude of tasks from patient physical care, to charting, collaborating with doctors and other healthcare professionals, comforting families, and even coordinating logistics like patient transfers. Prioritization helps manage this overwhelming load, reducing stress, burnout, and the feeling of fragmentation that can come from dividing attention between too many tasks.

A nurse who can prioritize effectively experiences more control over their work environment. They are more likely to feel accomplished at the end of their shift, having focused on tasks based on their urgency and importance. This provides a sense of purpose and job satisfaction - significant factors affecting nurse retention in the profession.

## 4.3. Prioritization and Healthcare System Efficiency

The efficiency and effectiveness of any healthcare system largely rely on how well nurses can prioritize. With better prioritization comes more streamlined and optimized processes, less wasted resources, and a more efficient healthcare system overall.

Firstly, by cutting down on redundant and unnecessary tasks, prioritization allows nurses to focus on meaningful and impact-making tasks. This leads to better use of resources and increased productivity.

Secondly, it can help reduce medical errors. Prioritizing safety-related tasks can prevent errors due to rushed work or overlooked procedures.

Lastly, it positively affects the quality of care, leading to faster patient recovery times and improved utilization of hospital resources.

# 4.4. Strategies for Better Prioritization

Having understood the importance of prioritization, let's delve into how to improve this critical skill.

1. *Urgent vs important:* Urgency and importance are the two principles often used in classic time management. Urgency is determined by timelines and deadlines, while importance is determined by how critical the task is to overall patient care. Ideally, tasks that are both urgent and important should get priority.

2. *Use frameworks to prioritize:* Several nursing prioritization models exist to aid decision-making. For example, the ABCs (Airway, Breathing, Circulation) is a simple framework that can guide a nurse on what tasks should be done first.

3. *Plan ahead:* At the beginning of a shift, take some time to plan out your tasks and anticipate possible crises. Early planning can lead to smoother transitions and less time lost on unexpected issues.

4. *Delegate appropriately:* Delegation is a key factor in effective prioritization. Understanding what aspects of care you can delegate to others can free up time for tasks that need your expertise.

# 4.5. Training and Tools for Prioritization

Multiple resources exist to improve prioritization skills. Formal training programs, mentorship, learning from more experienced nurses, or simulation-based training are some traditional routes.

Today, many tools are also available to assist with this. Task management softwares, electronic health records, AI-based prediction tools, and more. These can help automate routine tasks, avoid human errors, and provide insightful analytics for continuous improvement in prioritization.

In conclusion, mastering prioritization is a continuous process, requiring regular refining and updating as you gain experience and as situations evolve. But the dividends it pays in terms of better patient outcomes, increased job satisfaction, and an efficiently running healthcare system make it well worth the investment. After all, the beating heart of a thriving healthcare system is the nurse's ability to prioritize effectively.

# Chapter 5. Integrating Technology for Enhanced Time Management

The advent of technology into the healthcare sector has marked a new era of efficiency, precision, and improved patient care. For nurses, who act as linchpins in the healthcare delivery system, technology unfolds a canvas where they can deploy time management skills more effectively.

## 5.1. Embracing Electronic Health Records

In the quest for timely documentation and efficient information retrieval, Electronic Health Records (EHRs) play a pivotal role. EHRs, a digital equivalent of paper records, document real-time patient data. They aid in the quick look-up of patient history, lab results, and prescribed medications. This saves precious minutes otherwise spent shuffling through stacks of paperwork, thus improving the nurse-patient interaction time.

Practicing structured documentation in EHRs can further enhance your time management. Make a point to document in real-time; procrastination might lead to memory lapses, thus hampering the completion of records. Using templates and auto-population features can also help reduce the time spent on documentation.

## 5.2. Utilizing Automated Drug Dispensing Systems

Automated Drug Dispensing Systems (ADDSs) streamline inventory management and drug dispensing, freeing up the nurse's bandwidth for focused patient care. They increase accuracy, reduce time spent on manual counts, and decrease the likelihood of medication errors, thus contributing to patient safety. Moreover, ADDSs that incorporate advanced biometrics for tracking provide an effective safeguard against drug theft or misuse.

## 5.3. Proficiency in Telemedicine

Telemedicine can bolster time management substantially. Virtual consultations can reduce wait times and expedite care provision, allowing for the nurse to manage their time more efficiently. Brushing up on telemedicine setup and protocols, learning how to conduct online consultations, and gaining expertise in online patient education methods - these are all steps towards adroitly incorporating telemedicine into your nursing schedule.

## 5.4. Smart Scheduling with AI Powered Tools

Artificial Intelligence (AI) has seeped into several aspects of healthcare, including nurse scheduling. AI-powered tools offer smart scheduling by incorporating shift preferences of nurses, patient loads, and skill distribution among nursing teams. By reducing unintended overtime and balancing workloads, these tools render nurse scheduling a more streamlined and less time-consuming task.

## 5.5. Leveraging Mobile Health Apps and Wearables

Mobile Health Applications and health wearables proffer an excellent platform to monitor patient health in real-time. They free the nurse from the constant need to physically check on patients for vital signs or blood sugar levels. Real-time monitoring and alerts not only save time but also aid in early detection of health anomalies, giving a headstart on treatment planning. Encouraging patients to use these technologies and educating them about the same also forms a crucial part of a nurse's role in integrating technology.

## 5.6. Incorporating Electronic Bedside Shift Reporting

Electronic Bedside shift reporting enables seamless transitions between shifts, saving considerable time in the handover process. Pictures, diagrams, and linked notes provide an interactive way to understand patient conditions. Accurate, efficient, and inclusive - these are the three pillars that hold up this methodology.

## 5.7. Implementing Barcode Medication Administration Systems

Barcode Medication Administration Systems enhance patient safety and streamline medication administration. Scanning barcodes allows for quick verification against patient records, reducing the chance of medication errors and adverse drug events. This modern approach saves time and adds an extra layer of protection for patients.

In conclusion, technology offers a myriad of opportunities to improve time management in nursing. Embracing modern tools and strategies helps in creating a smoother workflow, reducing errors, and increasing the overall efficiency of a healthcare professional. Commitment to ongoing learning, adaptable mindset, and digital literacy are the key attributes for a nurse to integrate and harness technology for superior time management.

# Chapter 6. Balancing Personal Well-being and Professional Duties

A nurse's work life involves a constant interplay between personal well-being and the demands of professional duties. A sense of balance is critical to avoid burnout and provide quality patient care. This chapter explores strategies and methods to strike this balance effectively.

## 6.1. Understanding the Interplay

The duality of personal well-being and professional duties for nurses is more intertwined than it seems at a glance. As a nurse, your physical and emotional health directly affects your ability to perform at work. A nurse feeling unwell or emotionally drained is less likely to provide the level of care a patient needs. Similarly, the stress and demands of professional duties can negatively impact personal well-being. Understanding this connection is the first step towards finding your balance.

## 6.2. Recognizing the Signs of Burnout

Burnout, a state of emotional, physical, and mental exhaustion, is a common issue among healthcare professionals. It's crucial to understand its signs, which may include chronic fatigue, insomnia, reduced efficiency at work, disengagement, feelings of cynicism and detachment from the job, and physical symptoms such as chest pains, heart palpitations, shortness of breath, and gastrointestinal problems.

If you often feel disinterested, disillusioned, or excessively tired, it might signal that you are on the path to burnout. Recognizing these signposts allows you to seek help, prioritize self-care, and adjust your workload or schedule.

## 6.3. Implementing Self-Care Routines

One of the most effective ways to counteract work-related stress and avoid burnout is by incorporating self-care practices into your daily routine. Self-care does not have to be time-consuming or costly, rather it can be simple activities that rejuvenate and uplift your spirit.

Physical activities, like regular exercise, yoga, walking or jogging can reduce stress and bolster your physical health. Healthy eating is also vital. Make a point to take meals at regular intervals and opt for balanced diet comprised of lean proteins, fruits, vegetables and whole grains. Maintaining a consistent sleep schedule is equally important as sleep deprivation can significantly affect your performance.

Mental and emotional self-care is also key. This might entail hobbies that distract from work-related stress, meditation, or mindfulness practices to promote relaxation, or maintaining a strong social support network to lean on during challenging times.

## 6.4. Asserting Boundaries

Asserting boundaries is a proactive step towards balancing your personal life and professional duties. Declining additional shifts, setting precise working hours, and limiting work-related conversations during off hours are examples of boundaries that can protect your personal well-being.

At first, it may seem difficult to enforce these boundaries but remember that it's an essential step towards personal well-being. Being assertive in communicating your limits demonstrates self-respect and professionalism. You're not refusing to help; rather, you're acknowledging your limitations to maintain optimal functioning.

## 6.5. Developing Time Management Strategies

Proper time management is crucial in nursing. The ability to manage one's time effectively leads to improved efficiency, less stress, and better patient care. Strategies might include prioritizing tasks, delegating responsibilities, avoiding procrastination, and utilizing organizational tools like electronic calendars, mobile apps, and to-do lists.

However, time management is not just about organizing your work hours. It also involves setting aside time for relaxation, hobbies, and familial responsibilities. It's as much about scheduling appointments as it is about penciling in time for a movie or a dinner with loved ones.

## 6.6. Seeking Support

No one is an island, and seeking support is not a sign of weakness but a demonstration of self-awareness. Support from peers, supervisors, or mental health professionals can provide the tools needed to better manage stress and burnout. Consider joining a peer support group or seeking counseling services. These resources can offer tips, coping mechanisms, and even an empathetic ear when you need it most.

Creating a balance between personal well-being and professional duties is not an overnight process. It requires self-awareness, determination, and continuous evaluation, but the benefits permeate both personal life and professional sphere. As you embrace this journey, remember to be kind to yourself, celebrate the small victories and continue striving for that harmonious balance in being a nurse. With time, you will notice improved resilience, better patient interaction, and an overall enriched professional experience. Remember, the goal is sustainability and not just short-lived success. Our next chapter will then explore how to maintain this balance over the long haul.

(Note: While asciidoc lists were not included in this write-up due to the narrative style, they can be added upon request.)

# Chapter 7. Diving Deeper into the Art of Multitasking

The art of multitasking is undeniably essential in the demanding, fast-paced world of nursing where there are constant demands on your attention and time. As healthcare professionals, nurses are always required to have an eye for detail while managing numerous tasks at once. Mastering multitasking not only increases productivity and efficiency, but also substantially enhances patient care quality.

## 7.1. The Meaning and Importance of Multitasking

The term 'multitasking' was initially coined in the realm of computer technology, representing the ability of a single processor to execute several tasks or processes concurrently. However, in a human context, multitasking refers to performing multiple tasks simultaneously, shifting focus between tasks or effectively juggling them.

In nursing, multitasking is more than just an impressive skill—it's a survival tactic. With multiple patients to care for, each with diverse healthcare needs, nurses must be able to multitask efficiently. The ability to successfully handle multiple responsibilities, anticipate the needs of patients, and navigate emergencies could potentially save lives and significantly increase the quality of patient care.

## 7.2. Components of Effective Multitasking

Effective multitasking in nursing isn't about doing more things at once, rather it is about managing tasks elegantly, choosing the right focus at the right moment. The key components of proficient multitasking can be mapped out as time management, prioritization, stress management, and maintaining accuracy.

*Proper Time Management*: An efficient nurse knows that proper use of available time is crucial. Time management is about making the most effective use of your time and working smarter, not harder.

*Prioritizing Tasks*: Prioritization involves ranking tasks based on their urgency and importance. Certain things require immediate attention, while others can be executed later. By effectively prioritizing, nurses ensure that they provide immediate attention where it's required most.

*Stress Management*: Stress management is vital because multitasking can often lead to stress. Mastering stress management techniques not only helps nurses to manage their workloads better but also has a positive impact on mental and physical wellness.

*Maintaining Accuracy*: In a field where precision is paramount, maintaining accuracy while performing multiple duties is essential. A minor error can have a detrimental effect.

# 7.3. Techniques to Enhance Multitasking Abilities

Developing multitasking abilities is not about being able to do everything at once, but rather it's about strategically managing tasks to ensure maximum productivity and efficiency. Here are some techniques to cultivate these capabilities:

1. *Adopt a Systematic Approach:* Having a structured plan for your shift and staying organized can go a long way in enhancing multitasking abilities.

2. *Use of Tools and Technology:* Making use of organizational tools

and technology can also significantly reduce the workload and help you juggle tasks more proficiently.

3. *Build Mental Resilience:* Mental conditioning exercises, such as meditation and mindfulness, can help enhance focus, sharpen memory, and foster cognitive flexibility-- crucial attributes of effective multitasking.

# 7.4. Tips for Successful Multitasking in Nursing

While the ability to multitask often comes with experience, there are practical tips that can enhance this skill:

1. *Documentation:* Consistently update patient files. Careful documentation is crucial for ensuring that no detail, however minor, is missed in the hustle.

2. *Effective Communication:* Clear communication is key in multitasking. From discussing patient's conditions with doctors to handing over the duties to the next shift, effective communication ensures smooth transitions.

3. *Incorporate Breaks:* Regularly interspersed breaks can help refresh the mind, enhance focus, and prevent burnout.

# 7.5. The Role of Training in Honeing Multitasking Skills

Formal courses and practical training sessions can help in enhancing multitasking skills. Simulation-based training sessions, online courses on time management, and stress management workshops are some of the ways to master the art of multitasking.

# 7.6. Conclusion

Nursing is a profession that demands proficiency in multitasking. The art of successful multitasking is less about doing everything simultaneously and more about prioritizing and managing tasks effectively. With proper training, stress management strategies, and using appropriate tools and technology, nurses can master this indispensable skill to deliver high-quality and efficient patient care. Remember, the ultimate aim is not just to manage many tasks simultaneously, but to do so efficiently and accurately, significantly enhancing patient satisfaction and care quality.

# Chapter 8. Proactive Planning: A Gamechanger in Patient Care

Nursing is a challenging and relentless field, making it essential for any healthcare professional to create a proactive plan to enhance patient care. In the fast-paced realms of medical institutions, seconds matter, and every minute saved can correspond to a major leap in a patient's recuperation process.

## 8.1. Setting up the Foundation: Understanding Proactive Planning

Proactive planning in nursing involves anticipating potential issues that might happen during patient care and concocting strategies to mitigate these risks even before they occur. It's akin to having a road map that guides a nurse through his or her daily tasks and routines, minimising unnecessary surprises along the way.

Much like its application in other fields, proactive planning in the healthcare setting reduces stress, mitigates mistakes, bolsters patient satisfaction, and maximizes efficiency. It's a pre-emptive strike against potential conflicts, complications, and challenges, giving a nurse more control in managing his or her time, energy, and resources in providing patient care.

Moreover, proactive planning stretches beyond mere task management. It encompasses physical organization, mental preparation, expanding of knowledge and skills, and even self-care.

# 8.2. Three-fold Dimensions of Proactive Planning

Proactive planning as an approach can be dissected into three dimensions in the nursing context. Each of these dimensions supports the other, aiming for a common goal: improved patient care.

1. Task Prioritization: Dealing with the constraints of time and resources, nurses need to discern which tasks need immediate attention and which ones can follow suit. Decision-making in this phase should primarily be driven by patient safety and welfare.

2. Preventive Strategies: This dimension capitalizes on a nurse's knowledge and experience, driving them to devise contingency measures against known problem-causing factors. For example, if a certain medication frequently causes allergic reactions, the nurse must have alternative options ready even before administering the drug.

3. Stress Management: Nurturing resilience against stresses derived from the working environment is key to maintaining a nurse's efficiency. Stress, if poorly managed, can lead to impairments in decision-making and operational performance.

# 8.3. The Art of Prioritization

Proactive planning begins with the art of prioritization. Nurses deal with a multitude of tasks daily, and it's easy to be overwhelmed, lose focus, and make costly mistakes. The key is to discern the importance and urgency of each task, leading to the effective allocation of time and resources.

The 'Eisenhower Matrix' is a proven tool in this regard. It divides tasks into four quadrants based on their urgency and importance:

1. Important and Urgent: Patient emergencies fit this category. These tasks demand immediate attention.

2. Important but Not Urgent: Activities like patient education, paperwork, and the like can be scheduled at the nurse's discretion.

3. Not Important but Urgent: Tasks like processing routine paperwork that require prompt attention but don't significantly impact patients' well-being fall in this quadrant.

4. Not Important and Not Urgent: These are tasks that can be delegated, like replenishing supplies or scheduling appointments, liberating time for more patient-centric activities.

## 8.4. Sculpting Preventive Strategies

The second dimension of proactive planning revolves around preventive strategies. It incorporates risk management practices, constant learning, and experience-gained insights into the daily functions of a nurse.

Preventive strategies need a nurse to be observant, flexible, and imaginative. An observant nurse takes note of recurring patterns and problem areas, leading to devising more effective strategies. Flexibility enables a nurse to accommodate sudden changes without getting deterred. Imagination promotes creativity in problem-solving and navigating through challenges.

## 8.5. Managing Stress for Greater Efficiency

Lastly, proactive planning addresses stress management, an often overlooked aspect of healthcare. Improper handling of stress can lead to exhaustion, errors, or even burnout. Hence, it's essential to handle stress proactively to maintain professional efficiency.

Effective stress management includes strategizing daily routines, incorporating regular time-outs for relaxation, ensuring healthy diet and exercise, and leaning on social support whenever needed. Emphasizing self-care in the plan can greatly improve a nurse's resilience and workspace productivity.

# 8.6. Bringing It All Together

Combining the dimensions of task prioritization, preventive measures, and stress management, proactive planning becomes a powerful tool in a nurse's arsenal. Planning and forethought can not only streamline daily tasks but also leave a momentous impact on patient care.

Incorporating these aspects of proactive planning into daily nursing routines paves the way for improved clinical outcomes and patient satisfaction. The striking balance between caring for patients and self-care leaves a nurse prepared to face daily challenges without compromising quality of care.

Proactive planning equips nurses to harness their full potential. It not only boosts efficiency and increases satisfaction among patients, but also enhances the quality of life of the nurses themselves. Truly, proactive planning is a gamechanger in patient care, setting the stage for the efficient nurse of tomorrow.

# Chapter 9. Communicating with Stakeholders: In Pursuit of Efficiency

In the dynamic world of nursing, communication is key to effectual healthcare administration. Through clear and precise dialogue with all stakeholders involved, an efficient nurse can greatly enhance patient care quality, save time, and increase her productivity.

## 9.1. Understanding the Importance of Communication

One of the foundation stones of being an efficient nurse is communication. Nurses serve as the bridge between doctors, patients, and other healthcare professionals. They coordinate care, relay critical information, and ensure all medical interventions are properly executed. Many studies show a direct correlation between effective communication in nursing and enhanced patient satisfaction, adherence to care plans, and overall healthcare outcomes.

Communication is a skill, and like any skill, it can be honed and improved. It is a necessity at the epicenter of nursing, and pivotal in the interaction with a wide variety of stakeholders in the healthcare environment.

## 9.2. Building Bridges: Patient Communication

The most direct and personal stakeholder for a nurse is the patient. Effective communication with patients involves more than relaying what the doctor has said; it's about empathy, understanding, patience, and creating a rapport that encourages cooperation and trust.

Understanding how to communicate effectively with a patient means not presuming knowledge or perception but actively seeking to understand the patient's experiences and emotions. Empathetic communication is a technique where active listening is employed to a patient's narrative, instead of dominating the conversation. The nurse communicates best by understanding the perspective of the patient about their health status, personal life situation, and emotions.

Learning to tailor communications to the individual patient is vital. This includes understanding and adapting to their communication style, level of understanding, and personal demeanor. It is often helpful to use tactical adjustments such as non-medical language simplification, providing written notes and post-visit summaries, and confirmatory feedback. This ensures that the patient understands and remembers the conversation, which is of paramount importance in patient compliance and satisfaction.

# 9.3. Facilitating Interprofessional Communication

Interprofessional communication involves creating a dialogue with healthcare professionals across all disciplines. This typically includes doctors, therapists, pharmacists, dietitians, social workers, and specialists.

The key to efficient interprofessional communication is openness, mutual respect, and understanding. It's important to be articulate in explaining patient matters using clear, non-ambiguous language and to listen carefully to the advice and instructions of others. For example, in handoff communication, being thorough yet concise in summarizing a patient's condition, treatment plan, and potential complications is crucial.

Using standardized tools, templates, and checklists can also aid in this endeavor. Structured handoff protocols such as SBAR (Situation, Background, Assessment, Recommendation) are proven to reduce communication-related errors.

# 9.4. Encouraging Family Engagement

Nursing practice isn't limited to the interaction between healthcare providers and patients; it also extends to the patient's family. Engagement with the patient's family can have a significant positive impact on patient outcomes and satisfaction.

Effective communication with the family requires a delicate balance of empathy, assertiveness, and tact, ensuring sensitive matters are dealt with in a caring and respectful manner. It is essential to encourage their involvement in the patient's care while being mindful of the patient's wishes and privacy.

Strategies like family meetings and inclusion of family members in care-plan discussions can improve this communication. It's also key to provide family members with regular, timely updates and clear explanations of any changes in the patient's condition or treatment approach.

# 9.5. Mastering Written Communication

Despite the increasing use of electronic health records (EHR) and emails, written communication remains a major part of nursing. It requires clarity, concision, and precision, both in writing patient records and interprofessional correspondence. This means using clear language, avoiding simplistic or vague terms, and being comprehensive but brief.

Using templates for documentation, writing patient status updates using structured formats like SBAR, and always proofreading before sharing documents are all habits that can contribute to effective written communication.

# 9.6. Injecting Cultural Sensitivity

Cultural sensitivity in communication is about treating every individual with respect, taking into account their diverse backgrounds, beliefs, and attitudes. This respect not only improves the patient-nurse relationship but also enhances the nurse's ability to provide effective care. It involves understanding the patient's perspective, acknowledging differences without judgment, and adapting communication strategies to appropriately meet their needs.

Increasing cultural awareness and competence can be achieved through educational resources, professional development workshops, and open-minded interaction with diverse patient populations.

# 9.7. Embracing Digital Communication Tools

Information and communications technology (ICT) tools can assist in boosting efficiency in nursing communication. When used effectively, EHR, telehealth services, patient portals, and mobile health (mHealth) apps can greatly enhance communication ability while freeing up a significant portion of time.

Selecting appropriate ICT tools, understanding how to maximize their features, training regularly, and adapting to technological changes are critical to effective use of digital communication tools in nursing.

## 9.8. Conclusion

Present within every area of nursing, communication is an essential skill nurses must continually refine. From interacting with patients and their families, coordinating with doctors and other members of the healthcare team, to efficiently taking and leaving notes—clear and effective communication is an absolute must. Hence, by understanding, practising, and effectively employing these communication strategies, any nurse, whether a novice or veteran, can enhance their overall efficiency in patient care.

# Chapter 10. The Power of Delegation in a Nursing Environment

Delegation is more than simply allocating tasks; it is about understanding the unique skills and abilities of your team and making the most of them to provide high quality care to patients.

## 10.1. The Necessity of Delegation

The proverb "no man is an island" is perhaps no more relevant than in the realm of nursing, where the effectiveness of a team can quite often be a matter of life and death. Working in a nursing environment means taking responsibility not only for oneself, but also for the assigned patients, and needing to work alongside a team of professionals with varying skills and areas of expertise. No single nurse, regardless of their talent or dedication, can act as a substitute for a well-functioning, competent nursing team. Burnout is a growing problem in healthcare, and those who fail to delegate are certainly not immune. Delegation is not an option in many nursing environments - it is a necessity.

## 10.2. Understanding the Concept of Delegation

Delegation, fundamentally, is about shifting the responsibility for performing a task from one person to another. In a nursing environment, this, quite naturally, needs to be done carefully and mindfully, with a full understanding of each staff member's capabilities and the needs of the patient in question. When performed correctly, delegation is a remarkable tool that helps optimize outcomes across the board, with patients receiving well-coordinated, timely care, and teams functioning in a more streamlined, less stressed manner.

## 10.3. Steps to Effective Delegation

Following a structured, comprehensive approach can make unfolding the process of delegation much easier. Here are the key steps involved:

1. **Assessment and Planning**: Start by gathering as much information as you can about the task, the team, and the patient. Review each person's skills, training, and current workload before choosing who to delegate to.

2. **Communication**: Clearly communicate the task, including its objectives, deadlines, and any relevant guidelines or processes.

3. **Verification**: Verify that the person understands the task and is capable of performing it. Ensure they comprehend the potential outcomes.

4. **Surveillance and Supervision**: Monitor the progress of the task regularly to ensure that it is being carried out correctly, providing guidance and assistance whenever needed.

5. **Evaluation and Feedback**: Once the task is completed, take the time to assess the outcome and provide feedback to the colleague.

## 10.4. Delegation Errors to Avoid

While delegation is a useful tool, incorrect application can lead to serious consequences in a nursing environment. Some delegation errors to avoid are:

1. **Over-delegation**: This often happens when senior staff delegate too much, leaving themselves with too little to do.

2. **Under-delegation**: In fear of burdening their team, some nurses might choose to handle more tasks themselves, which can lead to burnout and reduced personal productivity.

3. **Wrong delegation**: Delegating the wrong tasks to the wrong people can lead to errors and/or sub-optimal outcomes.

4. **Mishandling Accountability**: When delegating tasks, the responsibility for those tasks gets shared, but accountability remains with the individual delegating, who needs to ensure tasks are fully and accurately completed.

# 10.5. Key Skills for Delegation

To delegate effectively, a nurse needs to develop several key skills:

1. **Communication**: Nurses need to communicate tasks succinctly yet fully, maintaining clarity and transparency.

2. **Assessment**: Nurses must accurately assess the skills and capacities of their team members, ensuring tasks are given to those most suited to them.

3. **Leadership**: All delegation is a form of leadership, requiring an understanding of team dynamics and the ability to motivate and support team members.

By mastering delegation, nurses can provide more efficient, effective patient care, while managing their workloads and reducing the risk of stress and burnout. These concepts, principles, and strategies elucidated so far are markers on your roadmap to becoming an efficient nurse.

# Chapter 11. Patient Satisfaction and Its Connection to Efficient Nursing

Patient satisfaction serves as an essential indicator in measuring the efficacy of patient care. Fundamentally, it reflects the extent to which a patient's expectations about healthcare services have been met.

## 11.1. The Implications of Patient Satisfaction

Patient satisfaction is not just about making patients happy with their current situation. Rather, it's about ensuring their overall health outcomes and instilling in patients the confidence to manage their health situation independently. High levels of patient satisfaction often equate to better patient compliance to recommended treatments, improved clinical outcomes, and reduced rates of hospital readmissions, emergency department visits, and delayed care-seeking.

Consequently, hospitals that emphasize patient satisfaction tend to have lower healthcare costs. By fostering relationships built on trust, empathy, and communication, nurses play an indispensable role in promoting patient satisfaction.

## 11.2. The Role of Nurses in Patient Satisfaction

Nurses often serve as the principal point of contact for patients, promoting a clear understanding of their conditions, treatments, and care plan. Effective communication is key to these relationships, significantly influencing patient satisfaction rates.

Addressing concerns promptly, displaying an empathetic attitude, ensuring patients understand their condition and treatment and involving them in decision-making processes are primary nursing responsibilities that directly impact patient satisfaction. By mastering these skills, nurses can significantly contribute to overall patient satisfaction.

## 11.3. Good Time Management Equals Better Patient Care

One crucial aspect often overlooked is the role of efficient time management in improving patient care. By effectively managing their time, nurses can deliver prompt care, reducing anxiety and the perception of neglect among patients. It's simple logic - more time spent with patients equals better care and subsequently leads to happier patients.

Creating a schedule can help manage tasks effectively, ensuring all patients receive the care they need when they need it. Prioritizing patients based on their needs and condition can prevent adverse effects and improve patient outcomes.

## 11.4. Successful Nurse Stories on Efficiency and Patient Satisfaction

Let us turn our attention to several inspiring stories of nurses who have leveraged efficiency and time management to enhance patient satisfaction.

Consider the case of Nurse Carol. An adept ER nurse, she was known for her composure and efficient handling of emergency cases. One day, seventy-year-old Billy arrived in the ER with symptoms of a heart attack. However, the ER was experiencing a busy day, and response times were slower than usual.

Rather than giving in to the pressure, Nurse Carol quickly prioritized her tasks, delegated non-urgent tasks to other staff, and dedicated her time to Billy. She promptly administered an EKG, stabilized his condition, and continuously updated him about the care plan. Her efficiency in managing her time and tasks greatly eased Billy's stress and increased his trust in the care he received.

Similarly, Nurse Amy, despite managing a large number of patients in the oncology unit, implemented efficient time and task management strategies which allowed her a few minutes of quality time with each patient. During these moments, she focused not just on medical procedures but also on strengthening patient-nurse rapport. By showing empathy and ensuring each patient felt seen and heard, she heightened patient satisfaction.

# 11.5. Strategies for Efficient Nursing Practice

Integration of efficient time management strategies into the nursing practice can improve individual productivity and patient satisfaction. Here are a few strategies:

1. Prioritization: Identify critical tasks that directly influence patient outcomes and prioritize them.

2. Effective Delegation: Knowing which tasks to delegate can allow for more focus on patient-centered tasks, thereby enhancing patient satisfaction.

3. Task Batching: Grouping together similar tasks can increase efficiency and save time.

4. Stress Management: Nurses need to take care of themselves to care for others effectively. Regular breaks, proper rest, nutrition are integral.

5. Communication: Efficient nurse-patient communication results in better patient understanding, compliance, and improved outcomes.

Conclusively, an efficient nurse does not only manage time wisely but also provisionally impact the ultimate goal of every healthcare professional - patient satisfaction. Nurses that work on cultivating a balance between their workload and care time, along with building empathetic communication, are vital for the future of the healthcare sector.